OVERCOMING STRESS: Successful Stress Management for Moms

Table of Contents

Introduction

4. The side-effects of stress

5. The types of stress

6. Areas in your life where you may experience stress

   - Stress at work

   - Stress at home

   - Stress with your in-laws

   - The stress of being a first-time mom

   - The stress of raising children

   - The stress of having a spouse

   - The stress of finding mom friends

   - The stress of being lonely

   - Unemployment stress

   - The stress of sexual harassment

Section 3
Stress relief – overcoming stressors in our life

7. Coping mechanisms – good and bad

8. Successful parenting even while anxious

9. Healthy ways to relieve stress

OVERCOMING STRESS: SUCCESSFUL STRESS MANAGEMENT FOR MOMS

TYPES OF STRESS , CAUSES OF STRESS, STRATEGIES, TOOLS AND TECHNIQUES FOR OVERCOMING STRESS. HOW TO DEAL WITH ANXIETY DISORDERS AND WORRIES. HOW TO ACHIEVE EMOTIONAL BALANCE AND STABILITY FOR MOMS.

BY

ISABELLA NATHAN

Disclaimer

This book is designed to educate and to entertain. The contents are the sole opinion of the author. The author is not offering it as legal, accounting or other professional service advice. Although the author and publisher have made every effort to ensure that the information was correct upon publishing and at press time, the author and publisher do not assume and hereby disclaim any liability to any party, directly or indirectly, for any loss, damage or disruption caused by errors or omissions whether such errors or omissions result from negligence, accident or any other cause. The author or publisher will not be held liable for any physical, psychological, emotional, financial or commercial damages including but not limited to special, incidental, consequential or other damages. You should seek the services of professionals before making any decisions. You are responsible for your own actions, choices and results.

Conclusion

OVERCOMING STRESS: Successful Stress Management for Moms

Mothers are often likened to superheroes as they have an almost supernatural ability to work on multiple tasks at the same time. Constantly juggling home, work and family responsibilities, and having to be on top of everything all the time takes its toll, though. All too often, busy moms become overwhelmed and stressed by all that they have going on.

Through this book, we'd like to take you from feeling overwhelmed and stressed to being an overcomer in every situation.

"Happiness not in another place but this place, not for another hour, but this hour."— Walt Whitman

We will look at what stress is, what causes it, what it does to your body and mind, and, more importantly, how you can beat it!

Did you know?
Stress is a natural reaction – it is a normal part of life.
Stress evokes a physical, mental or emotional reaction.
Even positive things cause certain amounts of stress.

The natural purpose of stress is to keep us motivated, alert, and ready for any eventuality – particularly to keep us from harm.

Stress only becomes harmful when we face constant trials without any relief. When that happens, stress builds up and we begin to experience tension and eventually **distress** – which is a negative stress reaction.

When we are in distress our bodies and emotions are negatively affected resulting in an array of symptoms which we will discuss later in the book.

The great news is that we will dedicate a large portion of this book to helping you recognise and

overcome the factors and symptoms of unhealthy stress in your life.

We will use real-life examples of mothers who experienced everyday issues and how stress negatively affected them and how they dealt with stress and stress factors. We will also look at research findings so that you know and understand that stress is not something that will simply go away unless you put in an effort to adjust your stressors.

Divided into three sections for easy referencing, you will find the following:

Section 1
Facts about stress, worry and anxiety

1. A brief look at the difference between stress, worry and anxiety
2. The symptoms of stress, anxiety and panic attacks
3. Four common causes of stress
   - Fear
   - Worry
   - Busyness
   - Chronic ill health

Section 2
The harmful effects of negative stress

4. The side-effects of stress
5. The types of stress
6. Areas in your life where you may experience stress

   - Stress at work
   - Stress at home

> Stress with your in-laws
> The stress of being a first-time mom
> The stress of raising children
> The stress of having a spouse
> The stress of finding mom friends
> The stress of being lonely
> Unemployment stress
> The stress of sexual harassment

Section 3
Stress relief – overcoming stressors in our life

7. Coping mechanisms – good and bad
8. Successful parenting even while anxious
9. Healthy ways to relieve stress

Section 1
Facts about stress, worry and anxiety

1. A brief look at the difference between stress, worry and anxiety

Although they share some of the same symptoms, stress, worry and anxiety are in fact not the same. The similarities make it hard to tell them apart though. As we mentioned in the introduction, stress is a natural, trigger response which is usually short-term.

Stress is not 'all bad' as there are times when stress gives us the boost of energy or motivation we need to avoid danger – be that physical danger or simply avoiding the repercussions of a missed deadline.

Stress causes a fight-or-flight reaction in us. When met with a fright, the adrenaline that courses through your veins, as a result of stress, will cause you to stand your ground and fight or turn and flee.

Real-life example:
If you are absentmindedly crossing the street and you step out in front of a moving vehicle, the driver will hoot at you. The loud noise will startle you and causes an instant stress reaction. This forces adrenaline into your body which allows you to run forward or backward and avoid being struck by the car. The minute you are out of harm's way, your

adrenaline levels will drop along with your stress levels.

In another example, if you are walking in the park and someone tries to snatch your handbag, the adrenaline that is awakened by the stress of fright will cause you to hold tighter and possibly strike out at your assailant until he leaves, hopefully, empty-handed. Once again, when you are safe and your handbag is tucked under your arm, the adrenaline will leave as your stress level drops.

Both of these events may leave you trembling. That is simply a reaction to the adrenaline that surged through your body. In both of these examples stress was a response to a negative situation.

Anxiety, however, is what would happen if you held on to the feeling of stress after one of the above happenings and let the incident trouble you long after it has passed.

For example, back at the office, you can't focus on your work because the fright of nearly being hit by a car has left you too upset to think. Or later that night you are unable to sleep because the memory of having your handbag tugged away has left you with a prolonged feeling of distress.

Anxiety is triggered by stress but doesn't fade once the initial threat which caused the stress has passed.
What are the symptoms of an anxiety disorder?

- Excessive worry
- Feeling restless or on edge
- Fatigue
- Difficulty concentrating
- Irritability
- Muscle tension
- Disturbed sleep
- Exaggerated startle response
- Psychological symptoms like stomach complaints, headaches, or dizziness
- Physical symptoms like rapid heartbeat, sweating, shortness of breath, or chest pain

What is the best way to treat an anxiety disorder?

Therapy
Dialogue therapy helps people identify, process, and cope with their anxietytriggers. Cognitive Behavioural Therapy (CBT) teaches people specific skills to target their anxiety triggers.

Medication
Most medication has side effects but can help alleviate the symptoms of anxiety. Medications include antidepressants, anti-anxiety pills, mood stabilisers, and sleeping tablets.

Lifestyle changes .

We will discuss this in-depth in the third section of this book, but there are home remedies like introducing daily exercise, eating a well-balanced diet, sleeping well and avoiding certain substances that may help you overcome the symptoms of anxiety.

What is the difference between worry and anxiety?

Using the words 'stress', 'worry' and 'anxiety' interchangeably is the norm, but they are very different. So while it's okay to be telling your colleagues how anxious you are about the new project you've been awarded, you don't want them worrying about you and your anxiety. Rather be straightforward and use the words in their context. In so doing you can assure them that you are experiencing a healthy form of stress that has you geared up so that you can mentally prepare yourself for the task at hand.

For your reference, here are 9 differences between worry and anxiety:

- Worry affects your head while anxiety affects your body
- Worry is specific while anxiety is generalised
  Real-life example:
  James is worried that he and Shelly might miss their flight because Shelly's anxiety about flying is causing her to experience a dreadful headache which is making it difficult for her to pack and get ready for the trip overseas.
- Worry prompts problem-solving but anxiety exacerbates problems
- Worry is often targeted at more realistic concerns than anxiety
- Worry causes mild emotional distress compared to anxiety

- Worry is temporary while anxiety lingers
- Worry is more controllable than anxiety
- Worry seldom impacts our personal or professional lives whilst anxiety most often does
- Worry is considered a normal state while true anxiety is considered a disorder that requires treatment

2. The symptoms of stress, anxiety and panic attacks

In this chapter, and for the remainder of this book, we are going to refer to 'distress' as 'stress' because of the colloquialism of the term 'stress' in the context of an emotion which feels like anxiety. Please bear in mind everything you have read up to now about stress being your body's natural reaction to a sudden change, and remember that stress in itself is not a bad thing.

The symptoms of stress (distress)
There are physical and emotional conditions associated with stress, for example; anxiety, depression, heart failure, strokes, obesity, stomach problems, high blood pressure, etc.

Before you experience the above conditions you may experience these symptoms:

- Frequent headaches
- Frequent illness
- Poor sleep quality
- Irritability
- Muscle tension
- Neck and /or back pain
- Feeling faint, light-headed, or dizzy

- Difficulty swallowing
- Sweaty palms
- Stomach problems
- Disproportionate worry
- Rapid heart rate
- Feeling overwhelmed
- Forgetfulness
- Poor concentration
- Low energy
- Loss of sexual desire

If you are aware of the symptoms of stress and you learn to use stress-reduction techniques you will be able to prevent the onset of medical conditions associated with prolonged exposure to stress.

The symptoms of anxiety
When you feel anxious, your body hits high alert and initiates your fight-or-flight responses. As a result, the most common symptoms of anxiety include:

- Feelings of panic
- Accelerated heart rate
- Hyperventilation or rapid breathing
- Increased sweating
- Muscle twitching or trembling
- Weakness
- Fatigue
- Difficulty focusing on anything other than the issue causing the anxiety
- Insomnia
- Stomach problems, like constipation, diarrhoea, or flatulence
- Avoidance of things that trigger anxiety

Anxiety may present itself in the form of a disorder like:

- Obsessive thoughts and behaviours; a sign of obsessive-compulsive disorder (OCD)
- Anxiety-related to a specific event or experience that may indicate post-traumatic stress disorder (PTSD)

The symptoms of a panic attack
A panic attack is an abrupt state of distress or fear

that climaxes in minutes and includes at least four of these symptoms too:

- Heart palpitations
- Severe sweating
- Getting cold or hot
- Shortness of breath or feeling smothered
- Feeling like you're choking
- Trembling or shaking
- Tingling sensations or numbness

- Tightness in your chest or chest pains
- Stomach problems
- Feeling faint, dizzy or light-headed
- Depersonalization - feeling detached from oneself or reality
- Fear of losing control or going crazy
- Fear of dying

Because of the severity of some of these symptoms, people suffering from a panic attack may rush to the hospital because they believe they are experiencing a life-threatening condition.

3.   Four typical causes of stress (distress)

Everyone has stress. It's a part of everyday life and, as we have ascertained, it is your body's natural response to a challenging situation. Sometimes stress is healthy because it assists you with a boost of energy, adrenaline, motivation or a cognitive spike that will help you through a tricky situation.

When there is no release or relief from stress it begins to take its toll on our bodies and minds; it develops into any number of physical and psychological symptoms or more serious health issues and disorders.

Fear

Along with worry, stress and anxiety, fear can often be misdiagnosed as either of the former because the emotions and symptoms are so similar. The difference is

that fear and worry are usually the results of a *known threat* whereas anxiety has no definable specific threat.

Real-life example:
Let's think about our walk in the park earlier where someone tried to snatch your handbag. A more accurate description of the stress emotion you would have felt in that instance is 'fear'. The threat was real – there was a real human being in your personal space; he may have had a knife or a gun. Fear, presenting itself as muscle tension, increased heart rate and quickening of breath, would be your body's natural response to the dangerous situation. Once the threat was over the fear would subside and so would the physical symptoms.

Anxiety, on the other hand, would cause you to feel these physical symptoms while walking in the park, thinking, worrying or imagining that you will be accosted, even though the threat is not real. There is no specific threat, but your mind has caused your body to produce adrenaline when it isn't necessary.

Fearfulness can lead to anxiety and an anxiety disorder will intensify fear.

When fear starts becoming unmanageable and interferes with your day-to-day life it is necessary to gain a deeper understanding of your condition. Excessive fear can be related to phobias, panic disorder or social anxiety disorders.

It is best to seek treatment because of all the negative health issues associated with prolonged exposure to fear and anxiety.

Worry

"Worrying is carrying tomorrow's load with today's strength- carrying two days at once. It is moving into tomorrow ahead of time. Worrying doesn't empty tomorrow of its sorrow, it empties today of its strength."— Corrie Ten Boom

Worrying is bad for your health. It subjects your body to prolonged periods of negative emotion which will lead to feelings of anxiety. Chronic worriers have revealed that they sense a constant threat of disaster. This leads to them becoming overly sensitive to their surroundings, turning every situation and each person into a potential threat.

This type of prolonged worrying can impede a healthy lifestyle by negatively affecting your relationships, appetite, sleep, and work performance.

Busyness

As moms, we are living increasingly busy lives; struggling to juggle work and home commitments.

Psychologist and author Alison Hill says this constant state of busyness is taking a toll on our physical and mental health. She goes on to say how the traditional 9 to 5 working days don't exist anymore because people are plugged into their devices even when they are not at work.

Too many people are overwhelmed on a daily basis, never feeling like they are accomplishing anything and therefore feeling anxious about their lifestyles. This anxiety has a snowball effect as it negatively affects our relationships and lifestyles, which in turn causes more anxiety.

Real-life example:
Do you think being a busy mom makes you successful or more important?
Ruth, a burnt-out mother of three, speaks honestly about her busyness. When I considered this question, and I was 100% honest with myself, I realised that being busy made me feel important. If I wasn't busy doing something I felt redundant. I very seldom took time to relax at home because I was afraid my husband or children would think I was slacking off. I volunteered for everything I was capable of at the children's schools and our church.

When moms in my circle of friends would meet up for coffee I often couldn't go because I was overcommitted. This would make me angry and resentful towards them. I would question why they don't DO more so that they would be just as busy as me.

I was a burden on my family because I would either make them help me with whatever I had volunteered for, or I was irritable toward them, or, even worse, unavailable for when they just needed me to be their mom.

The wake-up call came when I went to see my family doctor because I wasn't sleeping well, I was overeating, and extremely highly strung. She refused to give me medicine to treat the symptoms and told me straight-up; "You need to change your lifestyle".

It took several sessions of counselling for me to understand that my success as a mom was not dependant on how busy I was. My family needed me for who I was and not for what I could do for them, and if I didn't volunteer at school or church I would be giving someone else a chance.

I had to learn to say 'No' and take time out without feeling guilty. Six months later I am a far more relaxed person and everyone is benefiting from the less-busy me.

Chronic ill-health

After the initial shock of the diagnosis has worn off, you may need help coping with the emotional weight that your diagnosis brings. Living with a long-term health condition can make you particularly vulnerable to distress, anxiety, fear and worry.

Here are six things you can do to help you minimise the stress of living with a chronic illness:

Understand your condition

Learn whatever you can about the illness including its symptoms, treatment, stages, and prognosis. Don't avoid the specifics, ask all sorts of questions, and don't shy away from the negatives and the bad news. To fully comprehend, you have to be aware of everything that this condition entails.

Observe how your body reacts

How does it react to different stimuli? Take note of what alleviates or worsens your symptoms and make the necessary lifestyle adjustments. Keep a diary or jot down notes on a calendar and share your experience with your doctor or with others who may be walking the same path as you.

Trial and error

Experiment with different ways of managing stress and painful emotions. When you find a technique that works, incorporate it into your daily or weekly routine. Some ideas include:

- exercising
- stretching
- listening to music
- deep breathing
- meditation
- writing in a journal
- cooking
- reading
- spending quality time with family and friends

It may help to schedule time in your calendar for regular breaks and self-care.

Manage your life
Stick to your treatment plan. Take your prescription medication as directed and visit your healthcare practitioner as scheduled. Make daily decisions to include a healthy lifestyle wherever possible, for example; exercise may boost your mood and improve mobility, or healthy eating may ease symptoms.

Manage your emotions
Being diagnosed with a chronic illness is going to bring a score of emotions and most of them are negative; sadness, anger, fear, worry, anxiety, and depression, to name a few. Once again experiencing these emotions is a natural reaction to distressing news.

Experiencing these emotions is not the problem but *suffering* these emotions is going to make you miserable.

Your attitude will determine your quality of life. Develop a healthy acceptance of the changes your condition brings with it and this will help you adapt confidently to living within these constraints. Work on developing new skills and habits and take on a positive approach while you figure out what works best for you.

Manage your relationships
You might have limited energy and less time available for mingling and some people may not comprehend the health challenges you're facing. To save yourself from the added stress of strained relationships, make choices about where to focus your energy. Concentrate on the relationships that are most valuable to you.

Section 2
The harmful effects of negative stress

4. The side effects of stress (distress)
Distress affects our entire being and even has a ripple effect on those around us.

Cognitive side effects
 Anxious thoughts, reduced concentration, fearful anticipation, difficulty with memory.

Emotional side effects
Tension, restlessness, irritability, constant worry, depression, inability to relax.

Behavioural side effects
Sleep problems, difficulty completing assignments, avoidance of certain tasks, emotional instability, eating more or less than normal, taking up unhealthy habits like drinking or smoking.

Physical side effects
Tension headaches, stiff or tense muscles, grinding teeth, sweating, choking feeling, difficulty with swallowing, feeling faint or dizzy, nausea, vomiting, stomach issues, lack of libido, fatigue, tremors, heart palpitations.

Social side effects
Stress affects people differently, some people tend to withdraw during stressful times while others seek the company of others. The quality of relationships can be affected when a person is suffering from stress.

5. The types of stress (distress)

Stress can be divided into three categories.

According to the American Psychological Association (APA), there are three types of stress — acute stress, episodic acute stress, and chronic stress. Each of them has its own symptoms, duration, and treatment approaches.

Acute Stress
Acute stress is the most common and frequently experienced type of stress and is usually brief. It is the result of a reaction to a short-lived situation.

Real-life example:
You would be experiencing acute stress if you were concerned about a deadline that is looming, or if you are caught up in the emotion of the car hooting at you when you stepped into the street. The stress is in your head and is affecting nothing but your thoughts. Once you have met the deadline or you are safely back on the pavement, your stress levels will drop and your thoughts will settle.

Acute stress causes symptoms in your body, brain and emotions for a short period and therefore does not cause any long-term damage.

Short-term symptoms of acute stress:

- Any combination of anger, irritability or anxiety
- Muscular tension
- Short term elevation of blood pressure, increase in heart rate and pulse, sweating, shortness of breath, or dizziness

Acute stress is easily treatable and manageable.

Episodic Acute Stress

Frequent bouts of acute stress caused by having recurrent stress triggers present is known as episodic stress. For example, if you work in a very stressful environment that places huge demands on you, you may experience acute stress throughout the day. This is no longer just acute stress but rather episodic acute stress. This also applies to moms who have hectic home schedules.

Although the symptoms of episodic acute stress are similar to acute stress, because of their recurrent frequency, the prolonged effects will have a negative long-term impact on one's health.

Emotional distress

Anger, irritability, anxiety, short-temperedness, impatience, depression.

Cognitive distress

Difficulty focusing or concentrating, slower processing speed, difficulty forming new memories, mental fatigue.

Physical distress

Tension, headache, back pain, jaw pain, weakened immune system, stomach problems, high blood pressure, headaches, insomnia, chest pain, to name but a few.

Over and above these side effects, relationships are also compromised.

Episodic acute stress can lead to health issues such as heart disease, high blood pressure, ulcers, acid reflux and irritable bowel syndrome.

Treating episodic acute stress takes determination and professional treatment because the stress has become a habit and part of your lifestyle.

Chronic Stress

People suffering from chronic stress will need extended medical and psychological care that treats behaviours and promotes stress management.

Chronic stress upsets your whole body and can make functioning normally very difficult. Symptoms will vary from person to person but may include the following:

- fatigue
- irritability
- headaches
- difficulty sleeping
- difficulty concentrating
- disorganized thoughts
- digestive problems
- changes in appetite
- a perceived loss of control
- feeling helpless
- low self-esteem
- nervousness
- loss of sexual desire
- frequent illnesses or infections

Pay attention to how you react to a difficult situation and see how stress affects your life. If you feel you do not have the strength to cope and you are constantly overwhelmed, anxious, fearful or depressed, it may be time for you to seek help concerning a chronic stress disorder.

A continued negative response to challenges will harm your mind, body, emotions and ultimately the people close to you. Chronic stress is difficult, but not impossible to manage.

6. Areas in your life where you may experience stress

Stress at work

Stress isn't about an actual situation – it is about your reaction to the given situation. Work stress is usually caused when we feel we can't meet the demands on any given day or for a particular task, or project. Day-to-day work stress is normal and may even motivate us to work well and get the job done. This type of stress can be referred to as a challenge or positive stress.

Real-life example:
Teresa is afraid of speaking in public. She gets sweaty palms, her heart beats so that she's sure others can hear it, she feels lightheaded and struggles to swallow as her mouth is completely dry. Whenever her boss tells her it's her turn to speak at the next meeting she can't sleep the night before; she lies in bed going over what she has to say. Once the meeting is over and she has had a cup of tea to calm her nerves everything goes back to normal.

Other common causes of work stress are peer-pressure, the daily commute, deadlines, targets, and the like. When work stress occurs in quantities that make you feel like you're losing control, mental and physical stress symptoms may occur.

Stress at home

Healthy family connections are a source of strength that you can fall back on during times of stress. Family fun expands your fulfilment during the good times you experience throughout life. Conversely, an unhealthy family connection doesn't only deprive you of that joy and support; it can also create additional stress that robs you of your ability to cope. We cannot control the relationships we have with family members because they involve more than one person, but you can do things to promote harmony in these relationships, and in so doing avoid unnecessary family stress.

Dealing with difficult people is never easy, and just because someone is related, shares the same space as you, or – even more close to home – shares your blood, doesn't mean your relationship is going to be without challenges.

In this situation, communication and boundaries are your keys to mental health.

Stress with your in-laws

You *chose* your husband, but that doesn't guarantee that you are going to get on with his family. If you find visits or holidays with your family-in-law extremely stressful, here are some questions you could ask yourself to help you determine what the stressors are and possibly how best to deal with them.

i. Am I being overly sensitive?
    If you feel secure in your relationship with your partner and you have confidence in your abilities as a wife and mother, a little in-law stress shouldn't faze you too much.

ii. Do they have a point?
    No one likes to prod themselves too deeply, but if you ask yourself why their opinion matters so much, or if you are over-reacting, your honest answers may help you put the problem into perspective. You may not be able to change your in-laws but you can change the way you respond to them.

iii. Is it criticism or a difference of opinion? Everyone has their own point of view and if we can't share ours with our family, who can we share it with? Perhaps all that is different between you and your in-laws are your opinions on certain matters. Possibly you can simply agree to disagree without letting it make you anxious.

iv. Does my partner share my anxiety?
    These are the people your partner grew up with. They played a huge role in making him the man he is today. If he doesn't share your negative feelings about his family perhaps you should try and love them for who he is. If he shares your feelings then the two of you can work together on a coping plan of action.

v. Am I making a mountain out of a molehill? Most in-laws are ordinary people who are also dealing with their own issues and stresses. Unless the relationship is toxic you should work through your emotions and not let the occasional family visit or flare-up ruin your emotional health.

The stress of being a new mom

While preparing for the birth of your bundle of joy you imagine feelings of excitement, love and happiness – but what about the hard stuff like the fear of the unknown, adjusting to being a mom, struggling with emotions you've never felt before, lack of sleep, or guilt over longing for your old life back, even if for just a day.

There are few things in life as stressful as being a parent – and being a first-time mom must be in the top-five. Here's a look at some of the things that stress new moms out the most and some tips that may help you overcome the stress before it overtakes you.

i. ***Resentment***

... closely followed by guilt over feeling resentful. Don't beat yourself up about feeling this way – it happens to every new mom. Being the mother of a newborn is a 24-hour job and it's extremely taxing. Accept that there are going to be days where you don't feel warm and fuzzy about being a mom, but know that this exhausting time will pass.

Real-life example:
Kate, first-time mom, tells of the time her childbirth instructor drew a pie chart representing an 80-year life-span. Different colour slices represented different stages of our lives; school, college, marriage, etc. In the pie was a tiny sliver which represented our child's first year. "The point is – my baby is only a baby for 12 months. This truth helped me not to wish away my baby's first year, no matter how difficult it got."

ii. ***Sleep deprivation***

One of life's anomalies is that sleep deprivation causes stress and stress causes sleeping problems. Add to that a newborn with irregular sleeping habits and you have a recipe for disaster. But don't stress! That's why we wrote this book.

There are several ways you can work around the lack of sleep. You are sure to find one that works for you: sleep while your baby sleeps, take night-shift turns with your partner, ask your partner to babysit early in the morning so that you can sleep a bit later, or ask a trusted friend to come over and watch over baby while you catch up on some much-needed sleep.

iii. ***When baby won't stop crying***

When your baby cries it causes a natural increase in your stress levels; it's your body's way of getting proactive so you can prepare to solve the problem. But be aware that your baby can pick up on your tension – so if you are severely stressed this could exacerbate your baby's crying, causing you both undue stress.

When Baby cries, make sure they are not hungry, thirsty, wet, hot, cold, have a dirty nappy, or a wind stuck. Once you've checked everything on the list, and the baby is still crying, put them comfortably in their pram or cot and leave them for a while. The act of walking over to the window or stepping into the next room for a few minutes will allow you to gather your wits and remove any negative tension that the baby may be picking up on. Once you are feeling calmer, pick Baby up and try again.

iv. ***I don't know what to do***

Trust your instincts. You gave birth to the little bundle and you spend more time with your baby than anyone else. If something resonates with you, go with your motherly instinct before you reach out to family, friends, the internet or your doctor for advice. The more you practice your instinct the more likely you are to get it right and you and baby will grow and learn together.

Felicity, a childcare specialist, advises; "If your instinct turns out to be wrong, it's not going to have a disastrous effect on your child. Simply try another approach. What's nice is that you learn together. That's part of what builds the relationship between you and your child and makes you a stronger mother."

v. ***My house is a disaster zone***

If you can hire someone to help with cleaning once or twice a week that's wonderful, but if you can't, then I recommend that you treat cleaning your house the way you would anything else that needs to be done – prioritise the most important things and do them when you can. Once again, if you consider the big picture, your baby will not always be this demanding, your partner and your family and friends understand the pressure you are under, and if you ask, you will find they will be willing to help.

vi. ***Will my marriage survive this?***
The short answer is – of course! Millions of marriages have survived the first years of childhood and yours will too. It may be ironic to think that you and your partner created that little bundle that now seems to be pushing between the two of you. The truth is, your baby is demanding! Your partner is not. So you (both) have to put in a concerted effort to find each other amongst the chaos and confusion and make time for each other's needs. Try not to talk about baby all the time. Keep talking about your long-term plans and dreams. Make plans to do things away from home occasionally.

The stress of raising children

Being a mom is such a blessing – the bond between mother and child is so precious. However, being responsible for that little soul can create a fair amount of stress for moms. Most moms feel a certain amount of stress in some of the following areas:

Time

Finding the time to do everything that needs to be done every day is a daily struggle for mothers universally. Considering how many hats a mom wears throughout the day it's no wonder that we stress about not having time for everything, and of course, we worry if we spend too much time on other stuff and not enough time with our children. Then there are the odd occasions where we resent not having time to spend on ourselves.

Money

Your money stresses could stem from a loss of income if you decide to stay home with your children, or extra expenses like day-care or hiring a child-minder. There is also the cost of clothes as children keep growing and later the cost of schooling and extramural activities. We wouldn't trade our children for all the treasures in the world, but as mothers, we are subjected to financial stresses from time to time.

Relationships

You invest huge portions of your day in your children. As your children grow older they move from crèche to junior school and on to high school and you, as their mom, get to bump along with other moms who have children in the same stage of life. Family relationships and friendships that were formed before your babies were born may have to adapt and grow with your changing circumstances or they risk fizzling out.

As a mom, you may feel under pressure to maintain these relationships, or guilty when you feel you are neglecting others, or worse still, resentful about their freedom and your circumstances. Invest in valuable relationships, especially with your partner, your family and your long term friendships. One day when your kids are all grown up and leave the house you are going to be very glad you made time for these relationships.

The growing years

When they are little they want to put everything in their mouths. As toddlers they don't recognise the danger of climbing a wall or standing at the edge of a pool, as children and teens there is the threat of peer-pressure and social development, next thing you know they are learning how to drive a car and then heading off to college. It's a well-known fact that as our kids get bigger, so do the things we worry about.

Doubting yourself

As a mother, you have to make split decisions every day. There isn't always time to phone a friend when there are crises to handle, mysteries to solve and fires to pit out. Being under this kind of pressure is bound to take its toll and cause mothers to second guess their decisions from time-to-time. Am I doing a good job raising my kids? Am I too strict? Am I not strict enough? Every child is different so you can't do only and exactly what you read about or hear others say. Reviewing yourself as a mom is part of being a diligent mother, but don't become stressed that you are flawed and constantly making mistakes.

The stress of having a spouse

"Marriage is stressful by nature, even good marriages. It's easy to blame your stress on another person. Marriage is emotional weight lifting. It's

exercise. And when you choose to exercise sometimes it feels miserable. But the stress of parenting with a partner is worth it in the end." – Hal Runkel, therapist and father of two teenagers.

Many mothers feel stressed because their partner is not as involved as they would like them to be. From little things like allowing the kids to have a biscuit before supper, to larger things like planning the family's schedule, moms and dads think and do things differently because, although married, they are still two individual human beings.

Your spouse may not be helping exactly as you would like, but that is because he is not exactly like you. Allow your children to benefit from your unique parenting styles – provided they are not contradictory, because that will cause problems.

The stress of finding mom friends

Your children's age and their related activities will have you going to many places where you will meet other moms with children the same age. This is a great opportunity for you to meet new people and possibly make new friends.

This doesn't come without challenges though. It's easy to be surrounded by women who share a lot of lifestyle similarities with you, but can any of them become a true friend? One who won't judge you for feeding your baby food out of the jar, or one who won't feel inadequate when she discovers that you cook and prepare your baby's food from scratch?

Can you find a fellow mom whose style you are comfortable with and who will make time for you when you need a shoulder to cry on, or a friend to share a milestone with? Can you find someone who you feel comfortable with visiting you at home even when the house is a mess?

As women we feel we are being critiqued on our mothering abilities – or what we sometimes consider inabilities – and we ourselves may even be the ones tallying the scores in our heads. If you are stressed about finding like-minded friends you can be sure some of the other moms in your circle are feeling it too. Relax, you're all in the same situation and you're all doing the best you can.

The stress of being lonely

Alone-time can boost your mental state, but being lonely can harm your health.

How can moms be lonely you ask?

If a person who lives in the middle of New York City can experience loneliness then anyone can. Single moms who do not have the support structure of family and friends could be lonely even though they have a child or children to care for.

The long-term side effects of being lonely:

- An increased risk of depression and heart disease
- A greater risk of early death
- Increase the risk of contracting Alzheimer's disease

It may seem like I am stating the obvious – but the more friends you have the more social contact you will experience and the less lonely you will be.

Interesting fact:
social media connections don't alleviate loneliness.
People need real people in their lives to help them not feel lonely.
Too much social media interaction is known to exacerbate feelings of isolation;
it's as if our psyche knows it's fake.

Did you know that dogs can help you overcome loneliness?
Having a dog as a pet is sure to get you up and going in the morning and their antics will have you smiling. The companionship is real, and when you take your dog for a walk you may meet other people doing the same, and this brings a human connection to your life.

The stress of unemployment

Joblessness is a situation that can affect various people for a number of reasons including, companies downsizing, dismissal, health reasons, resignations, choosing to become a stay-at-home mom, etc. As with all stressful situations, everyone responds differently – some view it as a break from work stress or an opportunity to change career or explore different business options. Others struggle with the idea and it can lead to feelings of anxiety, anger, hopelessness or depression.

If you are struggling with anxiety over being unemployed, here are a few guidelines to help you keep your chin up.

- Don't take it personally; no matter what happened to cause your current state of unemployment.
- Accept your current reality. Once you accept it you move past the stages of anger and denial which inhibit you. Acceptance liberates you to move forward and start looking for alternatives or working with that you have.
- Establish a routine. Whether you are going to start looking for another job immediately, or if you are taking time to be at home with your children, establish a routine so that you don't feel unsettled by the lack of a work-day routine.
- Remember to have fun, just because you are unemployed does not mean you have to be miserable. Pick up on some old hobbies or start some new ones. One day, when you start working again, you are going to be sorry you didn't do more fun stuff while you had the time on your hands.
- Don't spend your days brooding about your situation. Questions like, "why me?" never got anyone out of a jam.
- Don't isolate yourself. Your family and your friends should be the first people you turn to. They know you best and will be able to help you deal with your emotions and show you how to think your way out of the situation. Join a committee or a church group if you feel you need more interaction. This is also a great way to network and meet more people who may help you get back into the job market or trigger a business idea.
- Focus on others less fortunate. Nothing will help you put your situation into perspective more than volunteering your time at a shelter for homeless people or abandoned animals.

The stress of sexual harassment

Unfortunately, sexual harassment is as real and it affects up to 60% of working women but according to a survey conducted amongst women, 90% of them will not report the harassment for fear of further reprisals or even job loss. *Source: 2016 EEOC Select Task Force on the Study of Harassment in the Workplace.*

The root of sexual harassment is more about power than sexual charm. Although a few exchanges may be the result of misunderstanding sexual interest; harassers are mostly busy asserting power over others. Women in authority are targeted because the harasser is using sexual allusions to belittle her authority. Men in authority harass women using threats of job loss or promises of promotion to try and win sexual favours. The harasser's aim is usually to humiliate and demean the person being targeted.

The symptoms of sexual harassment range from diminished self-esteem, to depression, sleep problems and anxiety disorders. Sexual harassment also negatively impacts the workplace dynamics, undermining employee morale and causing a drop in productivity.

There are systems and laws in place to protect women in these situations. Don't allow someone else's treatment of you to have a long-lasting impact on your mental health. Take control of the situation before it controls your life.

Section 3
Stress relief – overcoming stressors in your life

We have established that stress is a normal part of day-to-day life and quite a natural reaction to any number of happenings. What is not healthy is when the symptoms of stress linger and begin to cause problems with our health and wellbeing.

In this section of the book, we aim to provide you with an abundance of stress relief guidelines, tips and ideas.

7. Coping mechanisms – good and bad

Isn't it odd how we all have to deal with stress but not many of us know how to cope with it? Our coping mechanisms are as varied as your personalities and temperaments, but unfortunately not all coping mechanisms are equal – some of them can be harmful.

We know we need to deal with stress before it gets hold of us and makes us unhealthy, but are we sure that the coping mechanisms we have gravitated towards aren't also bad for our health?

Healthy coping mechanisms

Surround yourself with supportive people
People need people. We weren't designed to do life alone. Sometimes talking about your day, your problems or your fears with a good friend is all the therapy you need. Friends who are willing to listen and talk things through may even help you figure out a nagging problem because of their input or perspective.

Exercise

Getting your body moving is an amazing stress reliever. We're not talking about one-hour gym sessions or pumping iron until you resemble The Hulk(ess). Take the stairs instead of the lift or escalator, dance while you clean the house, take your dog for a walk, play outdoor games like Frisbee or ball games with your children.

Real-life example: *Tina, a working mother with two teenage children. I have a desk job that requires long hours of number crunching behind a computer. I can't make mistakes because I'm working with other people's money. The stress really gets me in my back and shoulders and the immobility makes my knees stiff and sore. I work on the third floor and made up my mind to take the stairs every time. In the beginning, my knees hated me, but they have loosened up now. I also told the kids to start dinner so that every evening I can take our dogs for a walk around the neighbourhood. Not only has the tension in my shoulders gone, but I've lost a bit of weight too. And when I get back from the walk I feel so energised instead of my usual tired and grumpy self.*

Aromatherapy
Scents such as vanilla, lavender and lemon have a calming effect. Mix these oils in with your hand lotion; have them in a diffuser on your desk, or light scented candles when you're home. One way of calming your nerves is to breathe deeply – why not breathe and inhale aromatherapy oils at the same time?

Make space for joy and happiness
"If you carry joy in your heart, you can heal at any moment." — Carlos Santana.
What makes you happy?
Do more of that!

Prayer or meditation

Taking the time to pray or meditate builds your inner-you. Your mind is free of stresses when you focus on a power that is greater than yourself. Handing your troubles and cares over to the source of your inner strength helps you unburden.

Unhealthy coping mechanisms

Excessive alcohol or drug use

The keyword here is 'excessive'. Enjoying a glass of wine occasionally is not excessive. Substance abuse becomes a problem when you use disproportionate amounts to help you escape your feelings of stress. Continued use under these circumstances will lead to dependence and eventually addiction.

Indulging in unhealthy food

Turning to food for comfort will only make you 'feel' better for a little while. If, when you're stressed you choose foods high in sugar or carbohydrates and with a low Glycemic index (GI) you need to pay attention. When these foods have worked their way through your system you will experience a blood sugar crash on top of your stress – so you are actually aggravating your stress. In future when stress drives you to eat, rather reach for healthier, whole food options that will help you beat the stress. We will discuss this again a little later in this book.

Sleeping for longer than required

Oversleeping to hide from stress is a form of escapism. You cannot feel the stress while you sleep but you also can't deal with it while you're in slumber land. Sleep isn't solving your problem it is merely postponing the inevitable – your stressors are waiting for you when you wake up.

Retail Therapy

There is no harm in treating yourself to a bottle of bubble bath so you can unwind in the tub or buying the latest book by your favourite author so you can relax and read, but spending money on unnecessary items becomes a problem when shopping sprees are your way of dealing with stress. More stress is heading your way when you get your bank statements and see how your spending sprees have negatively impacted your finances.

Self-harm
Overly stressed individuals may resort to harmful behaviours in an effort to gain control over certain areas of their lives. Rather seek help immediately if you can relate to this, and call someone if you think that you may be a danger to yourself.

8. Successful parenting, even while anxious

Being a mother is a combination of the most rewarding and most stressful experiences, sometimes mere minutes apart. Raising your children while you are dealing with an anxiety disorder is even more challenging.

Real-life example:
Stacey, mother of an 18-month-old, has been diagnosed with social anxiety and is seeking treatment. As part of her stress management it is recommended that she accompany her husband, Simon and baby, Mike, on an outing at least once a month. For this evening's outing, they chose to go to dinner at a restaurant. Stacey feels claustrophobic between the other patrons and is struggling to control her breathing, trembling hands and light-headedness. She is watching Simon speak but is unable to comprehend much of what he is saying. She has her stress beads to fiddle with while she counts slowly in her head. Placing her order with the waiter went well, causing her to feel a little more at ease. Suddenly Mike starts screaming because Simon moved the salt shaker out of his reach. A healthy mom would need a moment to compose herself before dealing with a child in this situation. Stacey was already stressed to the max when a major stressor is thrown into the mix. Can you envision how anxiety would rob Stacey of her ability to parent successfully?

Refresher note:
Anxiety stems from a deeply held core belief that we are unable to control or resolve a stressor. This belief causes us to question our abilities, doubt a positive outcome, and overestimate a potential danger.

A mother's fears can negatively impact the lives of her children.

- A germaphobic mother may prevent her children from playing in public parks.
- A mother who has social anxiety and never leaves the house will rob young children of the healthy social structures they need to grow and learn.

- A fearful mother may discourage her children from having boisterous fun and thereby inhibit their playfulness.

So, how can a mother who is dealing with a very real anxiety issue successfully raise her children?

Here are a few suggestions:

Look after yourself first
Seriously, you are not much good to anyone if you are anxious beyond all reason. Take the time you need to keep your symptoms under control. Three basic needs of humanity are rest, nutrition and exercise – so no matter how bad you are feeling, make room for those things for yourself.

Make peace with your limits
Without avoiding your stressors completely – because avoidance isn't a cure – be aware of what triggers your anxiety and deal with these things accordingly. Some triggers can be anticipated and you can prepare yourself for them; some are unavoidable. When an unavoidable trigger rises before you, try and implement the next point.

Practice your coping skills
What are your go-to coping skills; counting slowly in your head, deep breathing, a few minutes alone? You know by now that when you experience an attack of anxiety you can't think very clearly. Practice your coping skills even when you are not anxious so that they become your default when anxiety levels start to rise.

Be kind to yourself
Every mother has a meltdown occasionally where we say and do things we regret – our children are not the only ones that have temper tantrums. You are doing your best in a very difficult situation – don't make it worse by berating yourself mercilessly. You deserve forgiveness and compassion from yourself too.

Don't go it alone
Share your feelings of anxiety with your health care practitioner and be open about your condition with your family and friends. You shouldn't be facing these kinds of symptoms without help – there is a healthy way out for you.

9. Healthy ways to relieve stress

"The biology of emotional freedom depends on getting your endorphins flowing and turning off your stress hormones. How you achieve this? Laughter, exercise, meditation and doing anything that makes you loved."— Judith Orloff

There are healthy ways to equip yourself to deal with stress and anxiety. Self-help, mental-fitness, stress management training, and therapy help many people cope – but don't neglect the root cause of your stressors and make a point to get to the bottom of them. While you are working through your stress triggers or anxiety issues you still need to function in the real world, so here are some things you can do while you are on the road to recovery:

Exercise
We have touched on this subject various times throughout this book – this just goes to prove how important and valuable exercise is as a stress reliever.

Placing physical stress on your body alleviates mental stress.

People who have embraced exercise as part of their daily lifestyle are less likely to feel the effects of stress than those who don't exercise at all.

How does exercise relieve stress?

- Exercise reduces stress hormones (like cortisol) and releases endorphins (happiness chemicals) which actually improve your mood.
- Exercise improves the quality of your sleep which also helps you further fight stress.
- Regular exercise promotes confidence in your body which improves your general wellbeing.

Exercise mustn't be a daily grind – so find something you enjoy.

Interesting fact:
Exercises like swimming, jogging and walking,
which include repeated movement of your large muscles,
are particularly good for stress relief.

Prayer and Meditation
We get so caught up with our stresses and issues that we begin to think we are all that matters; the universe revolves around us and our problems are far-reaching and unsolvable. Taking the time to shift our focus from ourselves to a higher power helps put everything in proportion to the universe and all of creation.

Learning scriptures or reciting mantras may help you overcome undue stress as you focus on the promise of the words instead of your anxiety.

"Peace I leave with you; my peace I give you. I do not give to you as the world gives. Do not let your hearts be troubled and do not be afraid." – John 14 v 27

Eat well, feel well
"Tell me what you eat and I will tell you what you are". – French proverb
The best thing you can do for your physical and mental health is to follow a diet full of healthy, fresh whole foods. A diet high in sugar, refined carbs, processed foods and unhealthy fats will not only lead to unhealthy weight gain (which causes a whole different type of stress) but it also leads to less than optimal brain function which will affect your emotional wellbeing.

Spend quality time with people you care about
This is another point we have mentioned several times; once again, because of its value and importance in helping you deal with stressful situations.

The sense of self-worth and belonging that you get from your network of people will carry you through tough times. Women, in particular, benefit from spending time with loved ones as this activity releases oxytocin (a natural stress reliever).

Interesting fact:
The effect of oxytocin is known as "tend and befriend"
The opposite of the fight-or-flight response brought on by stress.

Ease off the coffee
Coffee contains caffeine which is a stimulant also found in chocolate, energy drinks and tea (except herbal teas). If you find that caffeine leaves you feeling jittery or anxious you should cut back. Some studies

show that moderate caffeine intake is healthy, but everyone reacts to stimulants differently; so be aware of the side-effects.

Take vitamins and supplements
There are a few supplements that can help your body reduce levels of anxiety. Here is a list of the most commonly used:

- Omega-3 fatty acids
- Lemon balm
- Green tea
- Valerian
- Ashwagandha
- Kava kava

If you have a medical condition it is best to seek advice before taking supplements as some of them react with other medication or have their own side effects.

Listen to peaceful music
"Music has recently been seen as beneficial for depression recovery; however, according to research it does depend on the type of music: Classical and meditative sounds seem to be uplifting, while heavy metal and techno can actually make depressive symptoms worse." – effectsofmusicinquiry.weebly.com

Deep breathing

Stress symptoms often result in a faster heartbeat and quicker breathing along with all the other symptoms that activate your fight-or-flight mode. For this reason, consciously slowing your breathing can help activate your nervous system into a relaxation response. The goal of the deep breathing exercises is to focus on your breath, breathing in through your nose and out through your mouth. This helps slow your heart rate too.

It's okay to say 'No'
Not all stress triggers are predictable and we can't avoid everything that stresses us, but you can take control of certain areas of your life and in so doing limit the things that cause additional stress.

If you are feeling overwhelmed and someone asks you to do something else, say no. One of the greatest causes of avoidable stress is taking on more than we can comfortably deal with.

If you are struggling with a particular stressor and you can avoid it, then do so, by all means. Just don't forget that ignoring or avoiding your stressors is not the long-term solution to overcoming them.

Stop procrastinating

Procrastination makes us behave reactively when we try and catch up – this will cause unnecessary stress. Rather, remain on top of your to-do list by giving yourself realistic deadlines while conscientiously working down the list in order of priority.

Make notes

Writing down what is making you anxious is one way of organising your thoughts about the subject.

On the positive side, making notes of everything you have to be thankful for will help you shift your focus off the negatives for a while – and that's never a bad thing.

Live in the moment

Being mindful describes behaviours that encourage you to live in the present instead of dwelling in the past or fretting about the future.

"I, not events, have the power to make me happy or unhappy today. I can choose which it shall be. Yesterday is dead, tomorrow hasn't arrived yet. I have just one day, today, and I'm going to be happy in it." — Groucho Marx

Essential oils

Also known as aromatherapy oils, some essential oils can assist with stress relief, relieve anxiety, and improve sleep. Add the oils to your body lotion or bath oils, put them in a diffuser or burn them as incense or candles. The most soothing scents are:

- Lavender
- Rose
- Bergamot
- Vetiver
- Neroli
- Roman chamomile
- Sandalwood
- Orange or orange blossom
- Frankincense
- Ylangylang

- Geranium

Promote affection

Want to release oxytocin and lower cortisol and in so doing relieve stress? Kissing, cuddling, hugging and sex between married couples are all positive physical actions that rid us of negative stress chemicals.

Pet therapy

Having a pet to care for is good for you because it:

- Reduces stress
- Improves your mood
- Gives you purpose
- Keeps you active
- Provides companionship

All things that reduce anxiety.

Laugh more

"Six-year-olds laugh an average of 300 times a day.
Adults only laugh 15 – 100 times a day. Be six again."
 Laughter IS the best medicine!
It's almost impossible to feel anxious when you're laughing.
Did you know? The physical action of laughter relieves tense muscles.

Seek professional help

Therapy, counselling or psychotherapy can help you cultivate healthy coping strategies to overcome anxiety. Trained therapists can help you find the root cause of your stress triggers and help you work through the issues to reduce anxiety. You may be unwilling to follow the advice given by family and friends, but if a therapist tells you to try something you trust their advice because this is their field of expertise.

Important note:

Therapy only works if you are willing to make the necessary changes.
You have to work on getting better.

IN CONCLUSION

"Remember, most of your stress comes from the way you respond, not the way life is. Adjust your attitude, and all that extra stress is gone."

Now that we know that stress is a healthy, natural reaction to any number of events or happenings, we don't have to worry about it too much. Our focus should rather be on the negative effects of not letting go of the symptoms of stress; not getting a break from stress; and the unhealthy side-effects and poor health conditions that accompany distress, anxiety and anxiety disorders.

This book gives you guidelines about the difference between stress, worry, fear, anxiety and anxiety disorders. Consider yourself equipped with the knowledge you need to understand what is happening to your body; how to deal with the stress and stressors; and hopefully never get to a place where stress and anxiety rob you of enjoying life.

If you feel that anxiety already has a hold on you, follow our stress-beating tips and guidelines and soon you should be well on the way to feeling like a successful stress-free mom.